Thank *God*

for antidepressants!

11ᵗ Feb 2014

Dear Rachel,
Ahh the best for your
life's walk,
   In Christ
     Jane

Thank *God*

for antidepressants!

a journey to new beginnings

Jane Newman

authorHOUSE®

AuthorHouse™
1663 Liberty Drive
Bloomington, IN 47403
www.authorhouse.com
Phone: 1-800-839-8640

Published by AuthorHouse   09/19/2012

ISBN: 978-1-4772-3020-6 (sc)
ISBN: 978-1-4772-3019-0 (e)

Cover photo: Rose Newman
Hippo drawings: Ian Pentney
Broken Pot: John Maire
Other drawings: Christina Krüsi

For John

For my children

Ann
Paul
Philip
Audrey

And for my grandchildren

Héloïse   the thoughtful, kind flower-gatherer
Mélissa   the go-getter and sweet hugger
Letitia   the story lover and whale-rider
Joakim   the snuggle bug

And those to come

Contents

Introduction

This is not another book on depression.

There are already so many it can be utterly confusing. Neither is this my method of how to get out of it in ten easy steps.

This is my personal journey towards learning to understand depression and cope with the questions it threw up for me; in particular the question of anti-depressants, and subsequently identity, hence the title of the book!

So why share my story? In a nutshell, it is a book written not by an expert, but by one who is IN it. Not only am I in it, but I have found that my life has actually been *enriched* by the experience, painful, desperate and frightening though it has been at times. Being on anti-depressants is *not* the end of the story. So this book is primarily for you, whoever you are, wherever you be, who find yourself in depression and needing medication.

I'm also writing for all those husbands and wives, parents and children, and friends who have faithfully walked through the depression of their loved one even though they have not understood what they were going through, and have often been at a loss to know what to do to help.

I salute my dear husband, John, who has walked with me through all the times of darkness and despair. An ENORMOUS, TOTALLY INADEQUATE thank you to him. A heart-felt thank you to those others who have encouraged and loved me through various times of depression and crisis and accepted me as I am, as a *person*: especially my children Ann, Paul, Philip and Audrey—they are my joy; and then dear friends Dawn, Adrienne, Clare and Howard, Les and Sara, Helen and Alistair (now at Home), Pierre-Eric and Jacqueline, Denis and Mireille, Didier and Lisiane, Bernard and Isabelle, Olivier and Juliane, Susanne and Erika, and all my Wycliffe Switzerland colleagues, who are also very dear friends.

Thank *God* for the doctors, psychologists, and psychiatrists that it has been my good fortune to be able to turn to: Doctor Bonnafous, our family doctor in Abidjan; Doctor Manfred Engeli, psychotherapist; Doctor Cristina Heierli, psychiatrist; Doctor Cornelia Lenoir, psychiatrist, these three in Switzerland. You have not only given me your expertise, but also your respect all shot through with a down to earth faith in Jesus Christ.

Then, I owe special acknowledgement to a new friend, Danièle, a psychotherapist, who accepted to be my "supervisor" in the writing of this book. Her interest in it from the start was an enormous encouragement to me, indeed made me take it seriously! And just as I was realizing that if it was ever to happen, I would have to be intentional and set chunks of time aside for it, Danièle asked me if I had set myself any goals for getting it done. Thanks to her I started setting intermediate goals for finishing a certain number of chapters, which I would then send to her. She has held me to it, and also congratulated me when I reached my goals! Thank you so much to my other cheerleaders who believed in this project with me, for Claire, Dawn and Adrienne. You also made me take it seriously!

Thank you *very* much to those friends, who under pseudonyms, have agreed to let me include something of their stories. That has made the book more representative, and enhanced its ability to speak to others.

And on the human side, lastly I acknowledge my debt toward those who helped edit my work and gave me thoughtful and invaluable feedback along the way: to my daughter Ann, my son Philip, Adrienne, Philip, Dawn, Danièle, Charles, Clare and Manfred. And thank you, John, for all your work on the photos. You are such an important part of this book.

And last, but not least, a special word to God: *Without You, I feel sure that I would never have made it to where I am today. Thank you more than I can ever express for the measure of healing, peace and fulfillment to which you have brought me today.*

May my story in some way meet you where you are and give you a measure of comfort, courage and hope; and dare I say it, maybe even a smile? I do hope so. Blessings on you!

Jane Newman, August 16th 2012
La Neuveville, Switzerland, a tiny town between Neuchâtel and Bienne to which I have come to feel I belong.

Chapter 1
Into unknown territory

Depression—from Latin, *deprimere* 'press down.'[1]

Depression crept up on me rather like some cancers: its beginnings hidden in the mists of bygone days, invisible, perniciously growing until it burst upon me "out of the blue," sometime in early 1985. I was in Ivory Coast, West Africa at the time. I broke down, like a car, and ground to a tearful, anxiety-ridden halt. I was 32, married and mother of two children aged two and five.

Apparently this was not, in medical terms, a *breakdown*; but that is the word that best describes how I experienced it. Even the responsibility of breakfast towered over me like a formidable mountain. *Breakfast!* It seems hardly credible, doesn't it? Don't people do breakfast in their sleep? But that's how it really was. And then, hard on the heels of breakfast came lunch, and hard on the heels of lunch came *supper*. Every day, for four people, for whom I felt it my bounden duty to feed healthily. It was like being on a merry-go-round that's going far too fast and which has lost the stop button. Molehills became Everests, and moments of decision, particularly those like, "What on earth am I going to fix for lunch," became nightmares. If someone had given me instructions for each meal, "Cook this," it would not have been a nightmare. And in fact, that is more or less what my husband came to do; that is we planned meals together.

I didn't understand what was happening to me, and I certainly didn't recognise it as depression. That medical term didn't mean anything to me at all. The expression, "to feel depressed," was of course familiar and a part of my active vocabulary as it is with most people. But this was different. This was paralysing, bewildering and terrifying, particularly because I had no name to put on it and it had come from seemingly nowhere.

Looking back, I had had a few intimations of what was to come in my early teens, but they were not recognised as depression by our family doctor of the time. On one occasion, when I was about twelve, he merely told me to pull myself together and stop making a fuss over nothing. This made me feel guilty, stupid and very, very lonely. I was, at that time of my life, on holiday with my parents who were living in West Africa. The rest of the time I was at boarding school five thousand miles away in England, from age seven to seventeen. I realize with hindsight, that the doctor's attitude reinforced a default function I had already developed, that of burying my emotions and feelings. It was this habit which enabled me to cope with being away from my parents for eleven weeks at a time for those ten years of school. I was so unhappy I used to cry myself to sleep for the first few weeks of every term, right up to age 17, and I often woke several times in the night.

I would creep out of bed so as not to wake my dormitory companions and tip toe to the nearest bathroom. There I would run a little hot water in the bath for my feet, and fill two mugs of hot water for my hands, and sit there in the friendly light, waiting for morning.

I put on a brave face towards my parents and towards my dormitory mates and threw myself into excelling in everything: ballet, piano, cricket, tennis, pantomime . . . whatever was going. Years later I discovered an interesting fact in my reading of Doctor Paul Tournier's books[2] that orphans, both literal ones and those who have to live apart from their parents, often compensate by forcing themselves to excel in life. The ensuing problem, as I found, was that I had to maintain my high position, or No. 1 ranking, which was a very stressful place to be in.

Why did I not confide in my parents? The reasons I am aware of now are these—I knew that it was a sacrifice on their part to send me to boarding school; it was for my good, and I'm sure that they meant it to be so. I also knew that they really hated saying goodbye to my brother and me at the end of each holiday. I can still picture them standing on the tarmac and waving as the plane taxied off down the runway. On top of that, being brave was part of our family culture; you bore suffering heroically without making a fuss. For all these reasons, I didn't feel I had the right to add to their unhappiness by burdening them with the knowledge that their daughter was herself so unhappy. In fact, it didn't occur to me that there was any other option. Boarding school was the done thing for expatriate's children.

I had a further, much deeper rumbling in the underbrush, when I was a university student living in France. I have an inkling that this was in some way connected to my new found faith in Christ although I don't actually know if this was the main cause.

However, it probably made things more complicated because of my unconscious belief, at the time, that Christians should be victorious in all situations, and know all the answers.

I don't have a clear memory of how things happened; just that it was paralysing me and that I couldn't even pray. But I do recall most vividly how I got out of it! I remember in desperation telephoning the director of a girl's camp I had been on. I didn't know many Christians at the time and she struck me as being very wise and very loving, so I called her. She told me to just repeat the name of Jesus as often as I felt necessary, and not to try to do anything else. To my amazement within a short time I was much better and as I said Jesus' name, I felt like I was being carried home on his shoulder. It spoke to me in a subliminal way, as pictures do, of his love for me *whatever*. I didn't have to pay my way with Jesus.

When I married, aged twenty-six, I started working full time alongside my husband in a Christian linguistic organization in the Ivory Coast. Linguistic research, literacy and Bible translation were what we were there to do, and I loved it. It was disappointing to me that early on in my first pregnancy I had to abandon most of my work due to severe nausea. However, I knew this was only temporary and that after the birth, an event I was enormously looking forward to, I would be able to get back to language work; so I wasn't unhappy about it.

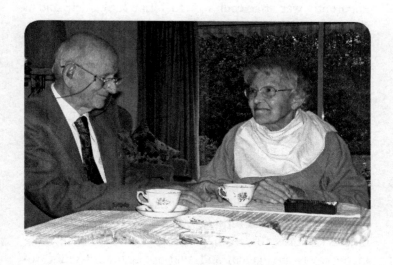

Complicity
Together through thick and thin—
on the day of Daddy's 90th birthday celebrations
in 2010

But then something totally unforeseen happened: instead of setting up home among the Jula people whose language we were to work in, my husband was to become director of the organisation's work in three countries. This changed the picture dramatically, because it meant that I would be "the director's wife" . . . a rather daunting and nebulous title! It apparently was up to each wife to define for herself, and as my predecessor was a brilliant and much laid back hostess, which I most certainly was *not*, it took me a number of years to shake off the unconscious drive to resemble her, and then discover what it could mean for me.

We were very young to take on this responsibility and at the same time to be starting our family: Newly married, new parents, and green missionaries—we had only been in Africa for two years—we threw ourselves into it, and paradoxically, those years were also the golden years. We had lots of fun getting to know each other (we had not actually spent much time together before marriage), each other's cultures (by reading special books to each other in our own languages) and sharing in the adventure of discovering life and new friends in West Africa. We had great colleagues, who were our closest friends, and they were the years when our family came into being and grew.

But the responsibility of director brought with it constant interruption and disruption of our family life, and frequent separations due to the amount of travel involved for my husband—echoes of the dreaded separations I had endured during my boarding school years.

I coped with these separations in the same way as I had coped with those from my parents; I dreaded them before they came, trying to be outwardly brave, and endured them when they were there, but deep down my feelings recoiled from them. Three years into the directorship we suddenly lost a very dear friend and close colleague; he died of hepatitis. The consequence was that his wife and three young children had to go back to Switzerland. We missed them all terribly, both as colleagues and as friends. The loss of Susanne was particularly challenging for me; she had been like an older sister, somehow her presence in our administrative and residential centre enabling me to cope with the times when John was away.

A few months later, still struggling to come to terms with this loss, I tried changing my malaria prophylaxis, my current one no longer being recommended; the result was an onslaught of three attacks of falciporum malaria in six weeks. That's the *bad* sort: Your head is so indescribably painful that you think it will explode. To treat it I was prescribed Nivaquine, which, among other things, gave me nightmares and bad nights. It was after those six weeks that things started to fall apart.

I became almost perpetually paralysed inwardly by anxiety and fear: fear of everything and everyone. I could no longer get to sleep at night, which made me more and more afraid of not sleeping, and you guessed it, made me less and less able to sleep. We found a solution for the initial falling asleep; my husband would read huge chunks of James Herriot's vet stories until I dropped. This worked fairly well, but I would awaken a short while later. I absolutely dreaded night time, listening to the peaceful silence of my family sleeping, while I fought conflicting thoughts, tried to focus on reciting Psalms from the Bible, only to be jerked awake each time I was on the point of dropping off.

The next morning, I might start thinking what a useless person I was, a drain on the family, spoiling their lives as well as my own and oh, if only I could feel a spark of enthusiasm for *something!*

And in the midst of all that, I would realize to my horror that lunch was coming round in an hour or two and my mind would seize up as I tried to think of what I could fix, and then supper would follow hard on the heels of lunch. Round and round I went, like being on the Big Wheel, with no way to get *off* it.

I remember being SO tired, so very tired from the titanic struggle to just survive and not go round the bend. Another lurch to the stomach, "Suppose I *do* go round the bend? They'll take me away from my family and I'll be put in one of *those* places . . ." Fear would then grip my heart and I would desperately determine to avoid that at all costs, but I wasn't at all sure I could.

To top it all, my hitherto normal sexual desire went walkabout. This regularly reduced me to profound mental crisis as I tried to bully myself into feeling desire yet at the same time realising that this was the most counterproductive thing to do. This was totally bewildering for both my husband and me. How could this happen, virtually overnight? That's what depression does to you, when it hits. Sex is the *last* thing on your mind. Worse, in spite of feeling affection and love for your partner, it isn't even on your radar screen.

How do you manage that? The thought of talking about it met with enormous resistance in me; it was so intimate, so threatening and dreadful in prospect. However, I am blessed with a husband who was more than ready to come more than half way to meet me. At various occasions, when I was particularly overwhelmed by the struggle, we talked, and he even got us laughing about it! This defused the situation enormously.

And I prayed. Over a period of twenty-five years I must have prayed the same prayer thousands of times. Many times I cried out to God because I was just so tired of *having* to pray to enter into something which had been completely natural. And I discovered a God who cared about me even to this very intimate extent. In fact, from my husband's point of view, we continued to enjoy a pretty normal married life. I made the decision to not talk about it all the time, for his sake, and to trust that God would come through in answer to my calls for help.

However, going back to that first time when things fell apart in 1985, the day came when my husband came to the end of his tether; he did not know what else to do to help. I mean, he was carrying everything, my load as well as his own. We *had* to get help; but where from? We felt at a loss. But suddenly a name came into my husband's mind, a missionary couple and especially the wife, Helen, who was a doctor. Both Helen and Alistair were so warm and welcoming to us, making space for us in their busy lives immediately. Although not familiar with depression they said they were ready to do what they could, God helping! Well, unbelievably, when we walked out of their apartment four hours later, my default function of burying my emotions and feelings had been brought to light. This has proved to be the central thing I needed to work on and indeed will probably work on for the rest of my life on earth.

I also went to see our family doctor whom I remember with affection. He was just so understanding and kind, and especially funny. Not about my condition of course. But he had this knack of introducing subjects into the conversation which burst the bubble of tension and made us laugh. He put me on to an antidepressant, the name of which I can no longer recall; after all, it was twenty-seven years ago, and I have no medical records with which to jog my memory. This enabled me to limp through to summer 1987 when we could go on extended leave and I could consult a psychotherapist. Enter Manfred.

My fortnightly consultations with Manfred stretched over a period of about 9 months, until just before the birth of our third child. It was my first experience of psychotherapy and I had no idea what to expect, but I was not disappointed.

One of Manfred's special phrases went like this: "most people try to do their best in life; it's just that they don't always know what's best!" I found this immensely liberating, from guilt as in, "I should have been able to avoid this. It's my fault." It also gave my self-esteem a boost, and was that needed! I had tried my best, but burying my emotions and feelings was not THE best. However it *did* enable me to survive.

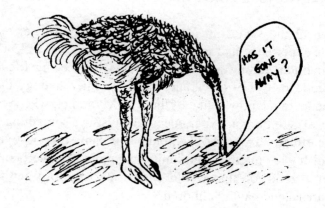

Burying—hiding from uncomfortable realities

As time went on, I was improving in the ability to spot it and stop it! I realised that it would probably be a life-long apprenticeship, and so it is proving to be, but I concentrate on the progress and not on the times I fail.

I was so happy at being able to come off the antidepressants; I felt a real sense of achievement. I had feared I would never make it. Once off them, I kind of vowed to myself, "never, ever again!" Not so much concerning the antidepressants, but the whole depression experience.

Yet, at the same time, I realized, to my surprise, that this experience had enormously benefitted me. I clearly remember telling people that it was like seeing life in colour instead of black and white. Another analogy that occurs to me now is that of the war. My father, whenever he talks of his war experiences, always says something to the effect, "It was *terrible*, but at the same time it saved me! It gave me the opportunity to get out of poverty and get a good job that would enable me to afford getting married and having children."

The next nine years went by with their usual lot of ups and downs, challenges, sickness,—mostly that of our children then—and so on. But some events stand out in my mind as being watershed moments; there was the birth of our fourth child after a pregnancy complicated with "pregnancy hepatitis." This birth was an unexpectedly healing moment in spite of the complications. Then there was our move from Ivory Coast back to Switzerland, with all the expected and *un*expected challenges that this threw up. Settling into Swiss life was hard for *all* of us, not just because we missed Africa so much, but also because of the cultural shifts that had happened in Switzerland during the fifteen years we had been away. It took quite some years for us to feel that were in any sense "home."

For John and me it also meant a change of job, although within the same organisation, and somehow living under a cloud of people's expectations, something we had not felt when in Africa. We also had the challenge of giving a considerable part of our time to helping the Church we joined in return for our rent being mostly taken care of. I in particular found these dual responsibilities to be heavy and conflictual. It felt like we were running two lives at once. Looking back, I can see that there were obviously issues there that were not being dealt with.

That being said, when I went to pieces overnight, after a period of nine years with no antidepressants, I was pretty devastated. This time we were in Switzerland; it was 1997, we now had four children between the ages of seven and eighteen, and were in the middle of moving house—just round the corner. One day I was thoroughly enjoying myself and packing up with gusto, and the next I was paralysed by anxiety, no longer able to sleep, and so on. Our family doctor prescribed Surmontil for me, which didn't help but gave me strong intestinal pains, so he referred me to a psychotherapist, Manfred again, and a psychiatrist. The latter was for the medication. Once again I was put on antidepressants, this time on Deanxit, one a day, and Surmontil on a low dose to counteract the over energizing effect of the Deanxit. Within a week I was feeling hugely better. The anxiety was greatly reduced and I was once again full of energy. And so I lived happily ever after? Not quite . . .

Chapter 2
Journey to the heart

*Votre raison et votre passion sont le gouvernail
et les voiles de votre âme navigante.*

*Your mind and your passion are the rudder
and the sails of your soul's journey. (My
translation)*

Khalil Gilbran, *Le prophète*

It is not easy living with depression. It is not easy to come
to terms with it and with the effect it has on one's family
and friends. And just when you think you've worked it
out, ping! Somewhere from deep inside there come those
doubts, those questions again.

It is not easy being on antidepressants either. I guess I had
known intuitively for quite a while that the antidepressant
I was taking, although in many ways enabling me
not only to cover the basics of life, but live a full and
interesting one, was not really the right one for me; but
I just couldn't make myself face it and bite the bullet to
change. Basically it made me feel *too* good, as in a bit
"hyper"; I had so much energy and so many ideas but I
didn't really have the strength to carry them out, and for
my husband it must have been, at times, like living with
a whirlwind! (*Amen to that*, echoes back!)

A friend of mine, also a psychotherapist, remarked that this was a case of "mood disorder". I had never heard of such a thing as being connected to depression. But it rang true, because for some time I had been wondering if my highs and lows, when on the Deanxit antidepressant, had a technical name. However, none of the psychiatrists or psychotherapists I had consulted told me that I was suffering from that.

But if you had asked me, back in 2008 or 2009, how life was for me, I would have probably answered "good, fulfilling, interesting, challenging, and fun". This would have at times been almost the whole truth. At others it would only be half the truth.

The reason for that, and this is what got at me most with this antidepressant, was a drop in my sexual temperature to below freezing. It almost sounds funny expressed in that way; but it was not at *all* funny to live with the assault it made almost constantly on my self-esteem and self-confidence. I felt abnormal, dysfunctional, out of sync, and lost. After all, it's not the kind of subject you can talk about in casual conversation. You need a very faithful, very understanding and close friend.

Late January 2010, I have no idea of the exact day, the doubts and questions were once again whirring round my brain as they had done periodically over several years: *I CAN'T put up with this anymore! Yes, I am leading a full and fulfilling life, but it's TOO full. And on top of that, I'm not sleeping well in spite of medication; it's like I'm being propelled through life at breakneck speed. And I want to give my best to my marriage. I need to give this priority and DO something!*

But I never seemed to have the recommended "quiet period" in my life in which to try this; it seemed hopeless. So I would convince myself yet again that I could live with it. It was so much easier to live with the inconvenience rather than leap into the unknown.

Then the words of my psychiatrist spoken two years previously would surface: *If you want to know whether you need antidepressants long term, the way to find out is to stop taking them for a while.*

This would be followed by the recollection of a conversation I had with a friend suffering from a different kind of depression, who at one point threw out: "You're so <u>lucky</u>, <u>you</u> can take antidepressants, and I can't". My immediate, unspoken, reaction was to think: So am I some kind of *fraud*, or what? My friend's lament unwittingly and unintentionally sparked off my identity crisis which manifested itself by the question: "Anyway, just who *am* I? Jane *with* the medication? Or Jane *without* the medication?" Or put another way, "Is the medication I'm taking making me into someone I'm not? Or is it, could it possibly and wonderfully be enabling me to be who I really am?" These are questions which, once raised, require an answer. They hit below the belt, and will not "just go away."

So finally, on that watershed day in January 2010, I stopped in my tracks, and looked the issue square in the face. "No! This cannot go on any longer; the questions troubling me must become my priority, and if my life is never calm enough to try this experiment, then I will just go ahead and stop the medication anyway, and that will force me into having to line up my life accordingly."

And that's just what I did. From one day to the next, I started reducing my main antidepressant to every other day and within a week to none at all. In my head I was convinced that what I had learned through psychotherapy during previous periods of depression was *sure* to enable me to manage just fine. But by the end of the week I was feeling really nervous, wheels spinning and "on the retreat" in life instead of "on the attack", and totally *spaced out*. My sleep was up the spout in spite of keeping on with *Surmontil*, which acted as a tranquilliser to counteract the super positive effect of the *Deanxit* I had cut out. I was not doing well at all. To cap it all, I was at a Church leaders' retreat; a small group of pastors, one pastor's wife and me, a missionary, meeting for the week-end to listen to God on behalf of the Evangelical Church at large in French-speaking Switzerland. Just imagine it! Listen to God? With nerves racked, wheels spinning, and a splitting headache, I was totally *incapable* of sitting still and listening to *anything*. The only thing I'm proud of is that I didn't try to hide it. I told these dear people, then excused myself for the rest of the weekend and either went out for long walks in the deep, fresh snow or helped with the cooking. It was the only way to stay sane.

I phoned my psychiatrist early Monday morning, between two trains on the way to work, only to hear an unfamiliar voice tell me that she was on a year's sabbatical leave and that she, speaking to me, (I didn't catch her name) was replacing her. She could take me—but not for two weeks. I was so taken aback that I said I'd think about it and signed off! *Idiot,* I remonstrated to myself; *you should have accepted the offer immediately. And you should never have started cutting out the antidepressant before seeing a psychiatrist. For Heaven's sake, why did you DO that?*

Yes, I did it all wrong and all I can tell you is, a far as it lies in your power, *don't* do it like I did it; just don't. And if possible, act *before* you get to the desperation point, because you are less likely to do stupid things like I did. But, if you end up doing what I did, get in touch with your doctor immediately.

What do I mean by stupid things? I acted both contrary to my own code of behaviour and to the advice of my psychiatrist. I was most definitely not in my right mind. Cardinal rule No. 1 says: Never, *never* reduce antidepressants on your own; only with medical supervision. I broke it, and now I was paying for it. And if that were not enough, I didn't follow the "reduction plan" given me by the psychiatrist; that little bit of paper stuck in with my pens and scrap paper. Now this is very humiliating to admit, because I can give you absolutely no rational reason why I didn't do it. Probably because my decision was in part irrational and arrived at in a moment of desperation. That's not an excuse, but an explanation.

On the personal side, I did the unthinkable thing of not discussing what I was thinking of doing first with my husband; he would have for sure pointed out to me that I must not start doing it without first consulting the psychiatrist. I was so convinced that it would be OK, and I wanted to "surprise him". Well, I did that all right, but it wasn't the kind of surprise I had intended, and it most certainly wasn't the kind of surprise he appreciates. Bad, *very* bad. I have since asked for his forgiveness and he has most graciously given it.

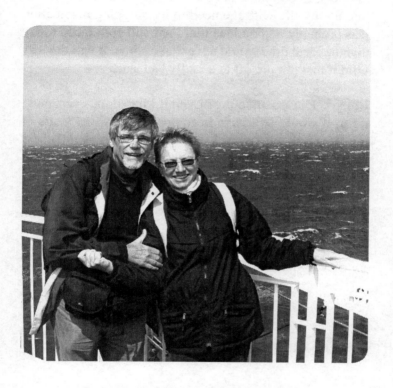

From North Island to South Island New
Zealand, holding on in the face of the Roaring
Forties—2007!
A parable?

However, there was *something right* in my intuitive jump into "the worst, and the best, year of my life": something *did* need to be done, and the decision to *force* myself to line up my life with the need to try stopping medication was probably a good idea too. I am still convinced today that the ideal time would never have come. It was the *way* I did it that got me off to a really bad start.

But you know something? Even if I had done everything right, it would still have been one of the worst years of my life. But the "worst" would have been slightly less awful at the beginning, and that might have meant that the worst was not quite so bad along the way.

However, I had unwittingly thrown myself into the deep end of a journey; I had set out on a pilgrimage to find out who I was. In more ways than one, it turned out to be a journey to the heart.

Chapter 3
On the slow train

*"If God had intended us to use aeroplanes, He
would NEVER have invented the railways."*[3]

On February 8th 2010, I walked into the consulting room
of the replacement psychiatrist and met Cornelia. And
I knew from the first that she was the right person for
me, even though she struggled a tiny bit with French,
being Swiss-German. Her caring attitude and ebullient
laugh that bubbled up from somewhere deep inside her
were infectious with hope. I felt respected as a person,
and although we had no first language in common, we
both managed with secondary languages, mostly French
and occasionally English when I was at my nadir of
exhaustion in body, mind and spirit.

Unfortunately, because I was about to set off for England
to spend a week with my elderly parents, I was unable
to start on a new antidepressant right away. This meant
that a whole month went by without the support of strong
enough medication, and my nerves were getting more and
more frayed, while my sleep was getting more and more
disturbed, less and less restoring. I would jerk awake at
4 o' clock every morning. At least in England, Bed and
Breakfasts provide tea-making facilities in one's room!
I drank numerous cups and did countless crosswords,
before I finally got up to start the day. Little did I realise

that my short nights would continue to worsen for another three months, racking my body, mind and spirit. Had I known that, I don't think I would have had the courage to climb the jagged, seemingly treacherous, soul-sickening, fog-enshrouded paths which brought me out, many months later, to my surprise, on to a sunshine-bathed mountain top where I could freely inhale the clean, crisp air and from where I could take in with a slow sweep of the eyes the true perspective of my surroundings.

But I didn't know, so, at the end of February I started taking a new antidepressant, *Mirtazapine*, on a low dosage. But by the third week, as the dosage increased, I was getting regular leg cramps, particularly disturbing at night time. So gradually we reduced the dose over a couple of weeks, and then towards the end of March, I started a second antidepressant, *Tradzadone*.

During the transition period I took temporary medication to at least get a minimum of sleep. Thank God for *Stillnox*! This gave me at least six hours of restful oblivion! I longed for this moment of relief when my head would hit the pillow and I would be "out" until four or five a.m. Unfortunately, I also started snoring very loudly which the French describe as *sawing logs,* which my husband endured with remarkable fortitude! I would then go and occupy our spare bedroom so as not to further disturb my him, and read, do crosswords, listen to music or the radio, and yes, you got it, make cups of tea.

This period of transition, coping with little relief for anxiety and jangling nerves, stretched out another month. I was still able to work, but finding it harder and harder to keep up the pace because of the prolonged lack of sleep and constant mental struggle. What kept me going was the thought that, come end of March, I would be starting on the *Trittico*, little dreaming that it would have a far-reaching and much worse effect on me. Ignorance is sometimes bliss indeed! I was also looking forward to the end of the month when we would start a ten day holiday. We hadn't planned anything ambitious, just doing day outings, cycling or walking, one of which turned out to be a moment to treasure.

It was to a nature reserve for observing birds. We particularly wanted to observe a pair of kingfishers that nested by a large pond. We were told that they never strayed far from the pond, flying from tree to tree on either side, or sometimes alighting on a branch sticking up in the middle of it. Three times we went into the hide and waited, and three times the bitterly cold northeaster drove us out after five minutes! We were about to go home, looked at each other and said, "Come on, let's try again!" This time we waited ten minutes and were handsomely rewarded. The kingfishers alighted on the branch jutting out of the middle of the pond and proceeded to put on a performance of a water ballet, and we saw it all from just five yards away. It was an almost prophetic moment to carry back with me to the daily round of struggle, with its subliminal message, "Be patient, you will see".

Actually, that holiday was a kind of oasis experience. My life was mostly like a dry, hostile desert, but I think we had sunny weather throughout the ten days, which meant we could get out and be physically active. This was one out of my bag of coping tricks: physical effort calmed my nerves and being outside lifted my spirits. Unfortunately, this was also to contribute to actually making things worse.

As the dosage of the *Tradzadone* increased I found myself feeling more and more nauseated. My psychiatrist encouraged me to persist, if I could, a little while longer because often these side effects disappear after a few weeks. So I continued, but because of the increasing nausea I was eating less and especially *drinking* less, yet pushing my body to do as much physical activity as I could—gardening, cycling, tennis; all in the unseasonably hot sun . . . By this time I was on full sick leave.

At my next tennis team training evening I nearly sprained my ankle from not moving quickly enough and found I couldn't focus properly on the ball. Hmm, I realised that I'd better cut it out, or it might be a broken ankle next time, or broken glasses. Things started to happen thick and fast after that. Three days later I started a urinary tract infection, and the next day an allergic skin reaction. So I was taking the nausea-producing antidepressant, antibiotics *and* antihistamines . . . In the end I pinned up a chart so that I could check things off throughout each day, it was getting that complicated! The last straw was to hear the doctor say, ". . . and you shouldn't go outside while it's the height of the pollen season." Not go *outside*? That was my *survival* tactic! That was like throwing away my crutches with a broken leg! Well, I started baking like crazy; biscuits, bread, cakes, anything to just *do* something and help pass the time, those endless, nauseas days that stretched out from morning till evening. I also contacted one or two friends and asked them if they would ever be free to come and play scrabble with me . . . and, bless them, they did!

But on the last Friday evening of April I just caved in over the kitchen counter, crying, "Lord, I simply can't go on any more, I just *can't*." In a kind of numbed state I somehow got to bed, so relieved to have the medication to help me sleep. And somehow I got through the weekend in a kind of daze, my husband's presence being of great help, of course.

After the weekend, Monday dawned, as it always does. John had gone to work and I was putting away the clean dishes and glasses from the dishwasher, and I was thinking to myself rather unintentionally that things really couldn't get any worse, that God had allowed every crutch that I could have leant on to be taken from me, when I became aware of a kind of peace deep down inside and then I started to think of Job.

Now Job is a character you meet in one of the books of the Old Testament of the Bible. He goes through a very, *very* horrible time. He loses his family, livelihood, friends and health, and basically would just like to lie down and die. He has absolutely no *idea* why God could let this all happen to him. As far as he could tell he had lived a compassionate, honest, upright kind of life. His friends tell him, "Not likely! You must have done something really bad or this wouldn't happen to you." Job answers them, "*Not so.*" Well, fortunately God intervenes at some point and tells Job's friends where to get off, and then has a private conversation with Job. He doesn't actually explain to him *why* he had to go through all he did, but challenges Job to realise that He, God, was in control even if it didn't seem like it. Then He restores Job's health, prosperity and family. And Job concludes, "Wow! *Now* I get it. I understand that I didn't really see God right before, now I see him a whole lot better." This is kind

27

of surprising, but on the other hand not. Job had been in God's washing machine, as a friend of mine once put it, with an extra long spin programme, and Job came out of it a profoundly changed man. My theological college Principal used to remind us that we can make suffering a minus or a plus. Job's combative honesty and yet respectful humility towards God made it a plus for him.

Now why am I telling you all this? Well, because as I thought of this man and his story, a very precise thought passed through my mind out of the blue: *this too will end.* I didn't need to find an interpreter to understand this thought that was given to me; from that moment I knew deep down inside that what I was going through had a meaning, even if it escaped me at the time, and also that it would indeed end. And that hope was like a lifebelt buoying me up through the month of May where I continued fighting the urinary tract infection with *five* antibiotics, and *none* of them worked. In fact, twice I was prescribed an antibiotic which was incompatible with the antidepressant and which gave me an even more unpleasant time.

Finally our family doctor said, "I can't give you any more antibiotics. If the infection doesn't clear up with this fifth one, you go to hospital." *What?* Now that was really *shocking.* At that point a friend who heard I was having a rough battle with the urinary tract infection recommended I do an Aloe Vera drinking gel cure, four dessert spoons a day for 2 months. Since John and I were on the point of leaving for England to visit my parents, I was only too happy to try *anything*, especially if it was a natural product with no known side-effects. Ten days later I had a urine test done: there was no more infection. It had gone![4]

But there was more good news. Back track to the beginning of May. With the psychiatrist we decided to slowly cut out the 2nd antidepressant that had made me so ill, and she suggested slowly starting a third one. At first I said, "No, that's enough, I'm giving up. Just let me go back on the Deanxit." But I am so, so glad I allowed Cornelia to persuade me to try. By the time I started the Aloe Vera, I had been taking the 3rd antidepressant for a couple of weeks and I was feeling *just fine.* No side-effects apart from a little putting on of weight (although this could also be due to much less sport and the digestive gastrointestinal candidiasis), no hyper feelings, and a *hint* of normal sexual appetite coming back. I could hardly believe it. As I write this today, I can tell you that things got even better. I feel my normal self, which is a pretty amazing thing to feel after years of *not* feeling normal. In fact for a while I experienced a sort of euphoric enjoyment of life, because it felt so amazing to feel well again.

For example, just eating my meals became a real pleasure, and funnily enough, my whole style of cooking changed too. I became a lot less tied to known recipes becoming very adventurous instead, with both successful and disappointing results! I'm sure that this was also enhanced by seeing the film "Julie and Julia" at about the same time!

And I had an answer to one of my questions: was I a long-term candidate for antidepressants . . . or not? Well, yes, I was, and I had learned that it was a chemical thing, not "all in the mind." That was so reassuring to hear.

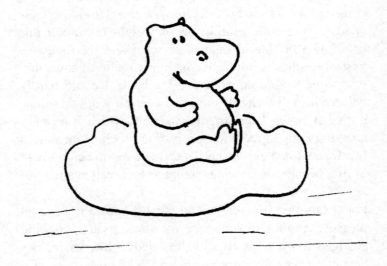

Cloud nine—feeling well at last[5]

Another thing that lifted my spirits no end was when Cornelia said to me, "When things were going really badly, I didn't need to tell you what to do, you *knew* what to do, and that's how you've survived this year.

But you need the antidepressants to enable you to *benefit* from what you know." That was about the most freeing thing I had ever heard. I felt like running around and telling everyone, *Hey, I'm OK, I'm OK!* It probably seems silly to you if you haven't ever faced depression, but *oh*, was it sweet for *me* to know! Even today, more than two years on, the wonder at feeling fully alive is still with me, although in a much less "over the top" kind of way. Of course, I was not only celebrating having found the right antidepressant for *me*, but also a recovery from the ill health that came as a consequence of the side-effects of the second antidepressant: no more urinary tract infections, no more hay-fever, gradually being able to cycle and play tennis again and so on.

But was I *really* OK? Or had I, through taking antidepressants, become someone else?

Chapter 4
To take, or not to take?

"We want no heroes here"

—Manfred Engeli

THAT is the question! Why *do* people make a federal case out of the question of taking antidepressants or not? You get all sorts of people giving their opinion; doctors, laymen, journalists, usually those who have never had to take them and have never suffered (to *their* knowledge anyway) from clinical depression. People get very hot under the collar about it and offer lots of gratuitous advice without any thought about the effect they are having on someone in their hearing who actually *takes* them.

The debate even featured on the Briefing page of *The Week,* 22nd October 2011, under the title of: *The riddle of antidepressants.* I was pleasantly surprised to find it a balanced, sensible treatment of the subject on the whole, presenting both sides of the question: to prescribe or not to prescribe? On the one hand, "an increasing number of doctors and psychologists are wondering whether they actually do any good . . ." and on the other, in the words of Professor Peter Kramer of Brown University: "There is plenty of hard evidence proving the benefits of antidepressants, but this is now being overlooked in a general shift of opinion against the drugs."

Jane Newman

The article then continues, to say: "The argument should not be about whether the drugs themselves work, it is about when they should be prescribed in the first place." It then mentions the Government's intention "to provide patients with a range of treatments that include both antidepressants *and* talking cures, or cognitive behavioural therapy, the latter with the aim of reducing the numbers of those claiming long-term disability benefit." Now, should it really be for *financial* reasons given that patients are encouraged to take a course of psychotherapy? I find this rather insidious and mercenary, and in the long run very short-sighted. What are the costs of caring for someone for whom you don't prescribe effective treatment and who has to be hospitalised? However I *do* approve the action of encouraging *more* than just medication. If you can stop taking antidepressants after a period of psychotherapy, so much the better! The snag is, as one doctor told me, that you often have to wait six months to get an appointment for psychotherapy. That's an incredibly long time when you're in a dark and desperate place.

However, to return to the question of whether antidepressants should be prescribed in the first place, you can look at it from an objective point of view, or a subjective one.

To take the subjective one first—If you're drowning, your head going under the water, far from land, and someone reaches down to grasp your outstretched hand, you will cling to it for your very life with no thought whatsoever as to whether it's the hand of a good person or not. Bottom line: you want out of there! That was certainly how it was for me. The questions of "whether I should," and "what if," came a lot further down the line. As far as I was concerned, there *was* no choice, period.

For others, who are not yet actually drowning, and who feel they possibly still have it in them to make it back to shore, the offer of the outstretched hand is to be resisted as long as they possibly can. They are able to take a kind of objective viewpoint, by which I mean, they can take enough distance from the dilemma to dispute the pros and cons, but often not enough distance to realise the state they are in. The famous New Zealand All Blacks rugby player, John Kirwan, makes the point in his landmark book, *All Blacks don't cry,*[6] that men seem to find it particularly hard to accept their need of antidepressants and indeed, to accept the fact that they are in depression. David Karp found in his survey, that people can even be taking off the counter medication, or someone else's prescribed medication, but they kid themselves that as long as it hasn't been prescribed *for them*, they're ok. Such is the resistance within many of us to taking antidepressants.[7]

From the objective point of view, I came to understand through explanations from Manfred and Cornelia that this is a complex question. It includes such aspects as:

- The reason for the depression: *external* (trauma, loss, family difficulties, loss of work, giving birth etc.) *internal* (the way I handle life and my feelings/emotions, missing chemicals in the brain etc.) *or both.*

- Whether to try a course of psychotherapy first, without medication, whether to start with medication only or whether to start the two simultaneously. However, not all doctors are sensitive to this issue or willing to explore the various options. In such a case it is important to realize that we, as patients, have the right to seek a second opinion. This could be too difficult to do alone. It's good to have your spouse or other relative or friend accompany you, as I did on one occasion.

• The state of the depressed person. Is there really a choice as to whether to prescribe or not, at least in the short term? In my case as mentioned above, when I first experienced depression, by the time I consulted a doctor I was in no position to choose. I took the antidepressants like that drowning person who clasps the hand that is offered to pull them to safety. It was much later, on the occasion of a relapse into depression that I started to think about the pros and the cons.

Let me share with you why I am *thankful* to take antidepressants, now that I've finally found the one that suits me for the long haul! I was glad that these same reasons were cited in *The Week* article I mentioned earlier because I think they are very important and often overlooked when people are discussing the subject "objectively". You guessed it; my reasons are all personal, and *sub*jective!

Firstly, they enable me to cover the bases! I can shop, cook and do the washing! On top of that, I can lead a "normal" life. By that I mean that, unless I told you, you most probably wouldn't guess I was taking antidepressants.

What's more, I can even lead a fun and fulfilling life! I can be on the offensive (though hopefully not *be* offensive) instead of the defensive; I have enough confidence to launch out into adventure, into new things. In other words, I look forward to most days as I get out of bed in the morning.

And last, but absolutely *not* the least, I can enjoy the sexual expression of love in my marriage once again.

The article in *The Week* was published partly because of a concern that antidepressants are prescribed in the UK far too automatically and without accompanying them with a course of psychotherapy, which can enable a person to understand how they got *into* depression and what they can do either to come *out* of it, or to cope *with* it. Now I resonate wholeheartedly with that. On the other hand, I would not want to see the pendulum swing to the other extreme and patients *not* receive the medication they need and which would help them benefit from the psychotherapy.

For many people including myself, antidepressants are like a plaster cast is to someone who has broken their leg. It enables them to get around, albeit painfully, (especially if using crutches), while their leg heals. The antidepressants enable people to be well enough to take a look at their lives, (the psychotherapy part,) then make some changes and incorporate new patterns that in the long term may well mean that the medication can be stopped. Or, as in my case, it may not mean that, but these survival techniques and new patterns have transformed my life so much, nonetheless, and enabled me to survive the terrible year of 2010 when I realized I wasn't on the right medication and set off on a six-month journey in search of the right one. Six months doesn't sound that long, but it was like six stretches of eternity.

But what are the objections to antidepressants? It seems to me that most are based on fear; fear of the unknown, fear of the known side-effects, fear of no longer being in control.

The problem of side-effects to antidepressants is a crucial one to consider, as with any other medication. If you unadvisedly read the little multi-folded, multilingual paper in your antidepressant box that advises you on all the possible side-effects you might have, you will find that the possibilities are virtually endless. (This is only a *slight* exaggeration.)They range from the quite tolerable, almost unnoticeable to the definitely *not* tolerable. And what makes it more complicated is that everyone reacts differently to them, whether in intensity, or in the symptoms experienced. So if I tell you that the one that suits me well and with which I suffer no unpleasant side-effects, is *Duloxetine*, this is absolutely no guarantee that it will be the right one for everyone else. It is a journey of exploration, occasionally excruciating as it was for me, but not necessarily so. And it should be, and for me it was, a journey done together with the psychiatrist. I think that my strength of resolve to persist was greatly helped by Cornelia's availability should I need to call "Help!" Even if she could not take a call right away, she would always get back to me as soon as she could. I didn't need to avail myself of that very often, but just knowing that I could if need be, was a great source of comfort and spurred me on to endure.

Now, the article in *The Week* makes the point that not all the side-effects of taking antidepressants long term are known. That's absolutely right. But *I* know what the side-effects are of *not* taking the antidepressants, and I know what I prefer to live with! It amazes me that this aspect is not brought into the discussion more often. Without it all discussion is lop-sided. In reality, I didn't have any choice in the "whether", but I could and can choose whether to accept the situation, or not. I have also chosen *which* side-effects I want to live with, and which ones I do not want to live with. Once again, I am extremely thankful that *Duloxetine* worked for me because it was the last resort. There weren't any more left to try. But I know that some people never find an antidepressant that could be said to suit them. They either have to put up with really difficult side-effects, or take nothing.

The fear of being "hooked" on antidepressants is also widespread, be it in the sufferer's mind or in what we read or hear. In my case, this produced in me the constant pressure to try to come off them as soon as possible. This was, of course, a self-defeating exercise. The more I looked to come off them, the less I felt able to. What helped me then, and subsequently, were the words of the psychotherapist, Manfred again, when I kept asking him "When can I stop them?"

"We want no heroes here. Don't rush to stop the medication. You will *know* when it's the right moment." And believe it or not, on that particular occasion, I did! These words calmed my fear instead of stoking it and released hope, and with it, patience to wait for the right time.

Maybe the biggest fear is that you will, in some way, be like a zombie or a robot. In short, you will not be yourself.

Let me tell you the story of my friend, Marion. She was a highly sensitive person who reacted to her environment and to medication far more strongly than would be normally expected. She couldn't stand any kind of noise, not even the normal noise of a few people talking in a room. She also suffered from many allergies and was hypersensitive to medication, and for this reason, she explained to me, she could not, and would not, take antidepressants. It was distressing to see this friend locked up into an ever tightening prison. I encouraged her to consider spending a few months in a specialised clinic, to which she recoiled in horror, as I think I might have done too!

Marion moved away from my little town so I no longer saw much of her. The news we got from her was not good though. Then one day we heard from her husband that she had been taken into that specialised clinic I had mentioned to her. I knew a little bit about the place as I had known the daughter of some colleagues who had had to go there. The first three months Ingrid was like a zombie, so heavily was she sedated. But, do you know? Within six months she was out of that place and able to slowly reintegrate her normal life. She never looked back! That was the reason I had recommended it to Marion, I was just so impressed.

So I was prepared to find her in the same zombie-like state, as indeed she was the first few times I called her on the phone. About 9 months later I bumped into Marion and her husband, who had come back to visit their friends in the area where I live. I couldn't *believe* my eyes. She was *radiant*! She looked *so* happy. And she had survived all that medication after all! I felt that I was seeing the real Marion for the first time and it was simply lovely.

Those nine months, however, were not plain sailing for Marion precisely because of her HSP condition. Each antidepressant that was tried gave her extreme side-effects; suicidal thoughts, manic depression with extreme highs and lows, and nearly drove her crazy. It was finally her local doctor who found the right medication, and in a form of drops that would permit very fine adjustments to dosage.

I asked Marion if it was worth it all, now that she is well. She answered emphatically, "Yes."

Now you who are reading might recoil inwardly in the face of her experience, which is understandable. Yet that would be to forget the crucial element of Marion's being a Highly Sensitive Person which added significantly to the complications of finding the right medication for her. It seems to me, that if we take that into account, her recovery in nine months is downright amazing. For me it spells HOPE.

Chapter 5
Breaking the taboo—
Facing up to attitudes

"Many, perhaps the majority, of those who go to see their family doctor have some type of psychological problem which makes them anxious or unhappy."

James Le Fanu, GP[8]

This does not mean that every one of these people needs medication for their psychological problem. What it does mean, to me at any rate, is that psychological problems are part of our human condition, but at varying degrees of severity and dealt with in very different ways according to the patient themselves and the world view of the culture they are in. Some cultures for instance, consider a person with psychological problems to be a crazy person. Our western culture did that too, not so long ago, and I'm not sure that it is entirely absent, even today—perish the thought!

What pleased me very much in *The Week* article already mentioned was that they quoted a famous person who takes antidepressants and who was willing to admit it! I salute the author, John Crace, for coming out in the public space with the fact that he takes antidepressants.

You see, so few of us admit to taking them! And with good reason!

You don't want to have people asking you every few weeks if you're better, however well-intentioned they may be. This puts incredible pressure on you to pretend you're fine when you're not, because their persistent questions make you feel as if you *should* be better.

Nor do you want to think that people are talking about you behind your back as in "she's got depression, you know," meaning "you don't want to take what she says seriously." This once happened to me. The effect on me was devastating. I cried inwardly for days and felt like all the stuffing had been physically knocked out of me.

Nor do you want to have well-meaning friends and family trying to put you right, as in "You just need to look more on the positive side, buck up, life's not as bad as all that, you should be grateful", and there you are just wishing "If only I *could*", or "How?"

I mentioned earlier the author, John Crace, quoted in *The Week* article. Here's what he has to say: "The professionally well might say I am deluded, that I am the victim of a medical conspiracy. Probably I am. But rather deluded than dead."[9] I'm not sure what he means by "dead" . . . committing suicide? Or experiencing living death? Either way, it's not a life. But hey, John Crace, "on antidepressants", is writing books! He's a regular feature writer for the Guardian on-line! I think that's fantastic. Thanks to the medication, he is able to give expression to his gift for writing, feel some fulfilment and satisfaction in it, I presume, and last but not least, earn a living!

Like John Crace, I have reached the point where I am ready to speak out to break the taboo, the hushed silence around the "D" word. I have come to realize that it's actually better for me to do this. It pulled the plug on fear of what other people think, and set me on the path of being "free to be". And it is a *path*; you don't change completely overnight, but the more you admit it, the freer you become.

However, during my first years of depression I was only at the beginning of discovering this was where I needed to go. I remember an incident, very early on in 1985. I was 33 at the time, and the mother of two children aged five and two. A missionary doctor, in whom I had regrettably confided that I was on antidepressants, immediately remarked: "You *must* come off those! You'll become addicted to them!" In plunged the knife of fear and panic and turned it another notch deeper than before . . ."I must come off them, I must . . ." but my fear had too strong a hold. Far from helping me, his remarks simply served to *tighten* the bars of my prison.

As a doctor you would have thought he would have known better, but there you are, none of us is perfect. I learnt from such experiences, and from the advice of my circle of trustworthy confidants, to only trust a few, select people with the truth of how I really was, and with everyone else I used what was to become *my survival tactic*.

The survival tactic enabled me to stave off the awkward questions, the worst being, "Hello, how are you today?" If anything was guaranteed to send me into a tail spin, that question was it! Until I realised one day that if I replied something like, "And you?", most people would not realise that I hadn't answered their question and would just carry on their way up the stairs or down the hall calling out "Fine thanks". And I was off the hook! That tactic was a life saver for me for *years,* because we were living in a large administrative accommodation centre for our organisation, so I was always bumping into somebody, somewhere, from the moment I stepped out of my apartment door, on the staircase, in the laundry room, at the sand pit where Mums and toddlers gathered, and so on.

On top of that, today there is opposition to taking medication in a much more general and idealistic way; it is in the spirit of the times. It has become the good thing to do to avoid taking medication if at all possible. Such influences affect us more than we realise, because they are largely unconscious. Nevertheless, the shame we can feel, and that I certainly have felt, is real.

These unconscious attitudes came to me through what I read in my women's magazines and were subtly communicated through people's general remarks and attitudes. And of course, in what was *not* said. It was, and as far as I can tell, still *is* a taboo subject in parts of many cultures today. I don't think people are conscious of it, and I certainly don't think they mean harm.

Yet there is no objective reason to hang our heads in shame. We are *not* second or third-class citizens just because we are *mentally* ill. Nor are we a drain on society any more than people with life-long conditions such as high blood pressure or diabetes are. Diabetes is a physical, objective pathology—lack of insulin. We could, as one doctor told me, say we are suffering from "serotonin deficiency syndrome"—a lack of serotonin. Of course, someone might then well ask: "What's that?" To which you could say, "It's a chemical lacking in the brain."

A friend of mine working in a Christian, residential, educational establishment told me her story. "Once my superiors knew I was taking antidepressants for depression, they reacted extremely negatively. This made me feel that I was suffering from a *shameful* illness. On top of that, they could not understand my need of medication. It was as if it were forbidden to have such a problem." Similar attitudes exist in the secular world of unemployment and work applications too, as another friend of mine was to discover over and over again.

It seems so silly that just by changing the label we put on something that it becomes acceptable or unacceptable . . . but that's how language works. Once a word, any word, has a certain negative connotation, chances are you won't be able to change that much, not in your lifetime anyhow. Correction, you can at least change it *for yourself*, and this may *start* changing it in other people's perception, by coming out and talking about it, openly and unashamedly. The more of us who do that, the more attitudes will change. But to do that you need to have processed the issue for yourself to the point where you don't care what other people think. As Manfred says, "we don't want any heroes here."

But that is the reason why I'm writing this book! Because I'm sure that, for all those who've told me they're taking antidepressants, there are thousands of you out there who haven't dared tell *anyone*. You may feel ashamed to be one of those "who go to the shrink", a nasty, derogatory phrase both for the psychiatrist and for you, and very revealing of an unconscious cultural attitude. Or you may be afraid of people's reactions and judgements, feeling awkward and ill-equipped to know just how to admit it, or how to field any remarks or questions that might arise.

Depression and the taking of antidepressants have a whole social dimension that penetrates all areas of our lives. It doesn't happen in private.

This is also true within faith communities. In some Christian circles it can be tacitly considered that Christians don't *do* depression. It's not so much a judgement or a teaching, as an unconscious, unofficial belief, which makes it all the more pernicious. Although I am thankfully not in such a situation, there was *one* Church member who, on learning that I took antidepressants, said to me, "Haven't you prayed about it?" The implication is that you ask, and bingo!

Happily, negative attitudes towards those taking antidepressants are becoming less prevalent. Indeed, the community I am part of is becoming ever less judgemental and ever more loving and supportive to those who in the past would have felt marginalised for whatever reason.

Indeed, they have been more loving and supportive than other friends that I have.

It was some thirteen years after starting to take antidepressants that I came to the point of being able to accept the situation; to accept myself as I was, *antidepressants and all*. This was in large part due to two loving and understanding people in whom I confided: one in England and one in Switzerland. And no, they didn't know each other! Their attitude was simply liberating. In fact, to me it was revolutionary! They both said, in the space of a few weeks, "Don't worry about when you can stop the antidepressants; just be *thankful* for them."

What was that? "Be thankful," they said, "that such medication *exists*." Now that was so much more helpful than worrying about if I should or shouldn't take them. There is power in thankfulness. And there is peace. I could concentrate on living.

It was about this time that I started mentioning the fact that I was on antidepressants, just in passing, and if appropriate, in conversations. Many people don't know how to react when you say it; they just ignore it, or just say "Oh." However I have never ceased to be surprised by the number of people who reply, in a low, conspiratorial voice, "So do I". And I sensed their conspiratorial relief to be able to say it! It's *that good* to know you are not alone.

And it gets even better when you can let go of the fear of others knowing. It doesn't mean you have all the answers, but you can walk tall.

Today, Lord, I feel like
a grubby, insignificant little earthworm;
things aren't going right, and I feel so stupid.
Everyone else seems so much nicer and cleverer . . .

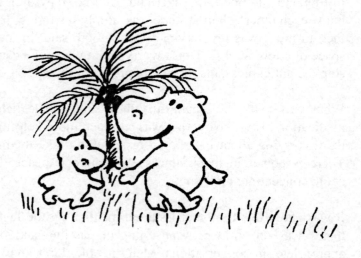

My child . . .
What matters is what I THINK OF YOU;
not what others think,
nor especially what you think about yourself.
I love you, today,
So walk tall![10]

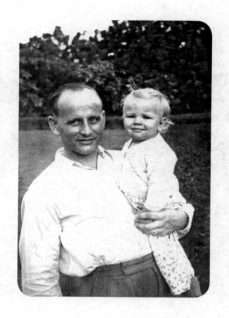

So proud to be with my Daddy!

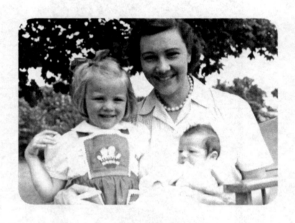

Aged 5, with my new little brother, Timothy

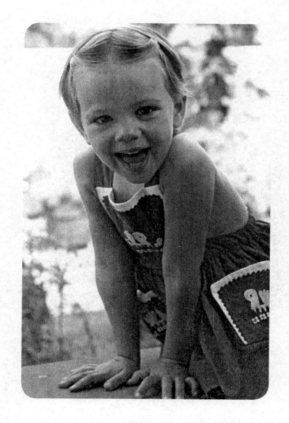

Aged 4, and happy in Africa

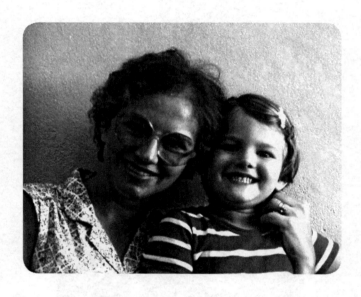

With my first born, Ann. Motherhood was a
wonderful surprise to me. To one who had
avoided looking after other people's children at all
costs, it seemed so natural!

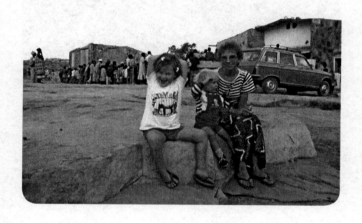

Just arrived in Sangha, in Mali, where the Dogon
people live, after an epic journey: 4 hours to do
the last 45 kilometres!

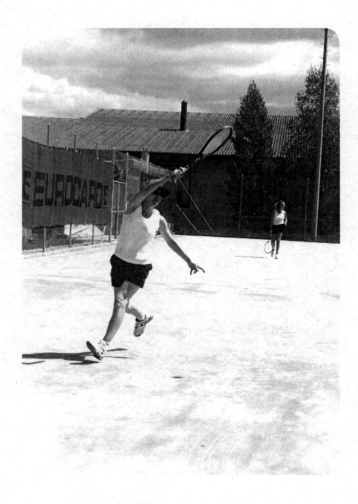

Playing for the "Young Seniors"
of La Neuveville. 2005
The enormous fun and dreadful angst of it!
Now I just do the fun part!

Chapter 6
In search of identity

*"You could not step twice into the same river;
for other waters are ever flowing on to you."*
Heraclitus, Greek philosopher
c. 535-c. 475 BCE

Or, put another way, you are and you aren't the same person with each day that passes.

So who am I? And does this really matter?

I would say that *anything* which causes someone existential angst is important, for the simple reason that they will get no rest until they've found some kind of an answer! Such questions grab your guts and refuse to let go. If you don't confront the question, chances are it will aggravate your depression. And of course, it's a question that your family asks about you, whether to themselves, or up front. Your children may ask themselves whether they are going to suffer the same illness . . . will they be like Mum?

I remember so well the moment in my life when I first was troubled by this question. We were living in our organisation's administrative centre, in apartment 17 which was basically a studio to which we had been able to annexe an extra room as a bedroom. My husband John had just become director, and Ann, our first child, was about eight months old. I was struggling big time with these huge changes to our lives. I felt very vulnerable, and haunted by the seemingly inevitable prospect that I might break down like my Mum had. It was like finding myself in a prison with no way of escape—condemned. I panicked.

I remember that as I struggled with this, a promise God makes to all who follow Christ, and which is found in the Bible, came to mind. "When anyone is joined to Christ, they are a *new* being."[11] (Italics mine.) I was in Africa precisely because I had "burnt my boats" and thrown my lot in with Jesus Christ. Faced with the question, "Am I condemned by heredity, to go the same way as my Mum," I gradually arrived at a place of trusting God's viewpoint: No I was a new creation. Nothing was *inevitable*. I might still bear resemblance to my Mum, but I was not condemned to live the same life she did. I was on a new path; I could get out of the heredity prison. While I loved my Mum hugely, my fear of having to go through what she went through affected my relationship to her for quite some years.

I don't recall ever being aware of Mum's struggles during my childhood years. I learnt much later that she had severe depression after the birth of my brother, when I was four years old. My memories start aged eighteen, when my father tried to explain to me that Mum was going through a difficult time. Settling back into life in England after twenty years in Africa was fraught with anxiety for Mum, added to which Daddy had started a new career and had to work extremely hard to get it going, and they had to start from scratch in making friends in the area they had decided to settle in so as to be near my brother's and my boarding schools.

Mummy died last year after a number of years with something akin to Alzheimer's. It was an opportunity to think back on my memories of her, but also to learn many new things about her from all the friends who wrote to the family. In my memory she was a champion picnic maker, whose salmon and cucumber, and tongue sandwiches melted in your mouth. She could be full of fun and quite cheeky, but at the same time so supportive and kind, when not bound by anxiety. A number of friends testified to her being a gracious and kind hostess to newcomers in the business community in Ghana, making sure that they were included in various activities.

She was an accomplished pianist, playing Chopin with great depth of feeling, and a good piano teacher. She could also have become quite well-known as an artist, if the few paintings she did are anything to go by. But in these areas, as in her cooking, which was brilliant, depression seemed to hold her back, undermining the little confidence she had.

I did not realize that it would take me many years to find the path to freedom, which in the event, lay within the parameters of hereditary frailty in the area of depression. But my pathway has been quite different from that of my Mum's. This may sound like the promise quoted above, "When anyone is joined to Christ, they are a *new* being," wasn't entirely true. But these words, in their context, are not talking about an instant transformation, but rather an instant transition to being a "work in progress", to being God's friends instead of his enemies, and also to being members of his team, involved in His work. The point the apostle Paul was making was that this is how we are regarded by God, and should be regarded by others; in a word, with *hope*.

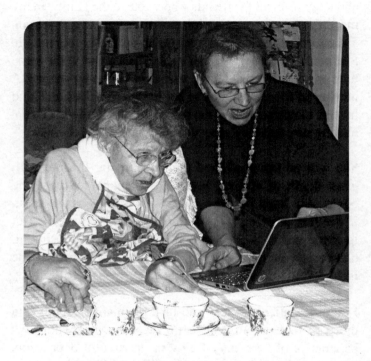

Mummy, just three months before she died

Ever true to herself, she is taking a keen
interest in my new "toy", bought with money
she had put by for me.

The first "post" along my path was to take on board that I was suffering from depression, that I was ill. From there I gradually learned to "make friends" with myself as I was, and not how I would have liked to have been. According to Professor Paul Gilbert, this is an essential step to coming out of depression.

The most important thing is for you to avoid feeling ashamed about being depressed. So, 'own' your depression and explore what you can do to change it or turn it off.[12]

Then, as the years stretched out from 1997 to the present day, I came to the second "post" where I had to "make friends" with the reality that I was not only mentally frail, but had a long term mental condition for which I needed to take *long term* medication. That was far more difficult.

But I think it is only over the past three years that I have had identity questions raising their heads connected with the long-term taking of antidepressants, which I have already mentioned in an earlier chapter. There were two main ones: Was I a cheat in taking the pills—*escaping* from who I really was? And, was the Deanxit medication the right one for me—that is, was it helping me to be whole, or was it in some way *distorting* who I was? The first question came as a result of my friend Marion's remark, but the second came from an inner realisation, or "voice" that gradually grew in volume until it was deafening me!

The questions seem to be quite different, but actually, I don't think they are, because they are basically asking, "Is it me, or my medication?"[13] And, "Who am I?" Now I cannot give you a medical answer to that. I have no medical training. But I can tell you the working answer I arrived at and something of how I got there. The path was both rational and intuitive.

On the rational side, the consultations with my psychiatrist, Cornelia were an enormous help. She explained to me that serotonin and noradrenaline insufficiency are observable, objective phenomena in the brain, not "all in the mind," as some people condescendingly remark. Special images of the brain of a person in depression can be observed, and then compared, before the start of medication, during and after it. The impact of this knowledge on me was profound. It swept away all feelings of being somehow "second-class", not up to the mark as a human being, and somehow lacking in my faith in Christ. It dawned on me that I was not to blame. I was not responsible for the condition. This did not, of course, preclude my being responsible to seek help for it. This was in one way, the real me, in the same way as if I had been born with a physical deformity, like a cleft palate; that would also be me.

What if I *had* been born with a cleft palate? Would my family, in the name of authenticity, have wanted or expected me to stay like that, ignoring the available surgical solution that would heal me? I don't think so. I think that when we see someone like that, and then see them healed after surgical intervention, we somehow think that *now* we are seeing the real person, as they were meant to be. We're really glad for them!

But when it comes to mental deformation, many don't intuitively see it that way, not even the mentally ill themselves. This may be for a number of reasons . . . Over the centuries, understanding of mental illness has lagged way behind that of physical illness. What we don't know we often fear and sometimes stigmatise. Mental illness is not visible to the unspecialised person, although the effects may well be. Cultural and religious world views also have great influence on how we see and judge things. And then there is the close link between the mind and personality. Does taking antidepressants imply personality manipulation?

All these reasons, and probably more, create the taboo and stigma around mental illness which lead it to being talked about in hushed tones and behind people's backs. This in turn feeds the identity crisis that many who take antidepressants long term find themselves in, at one point or another.

But now to the intuitive sense I had as to who I really was. This is, of course, totally subjective . . . but does that make it less true? Does that disqualify it? Not according to the sociologist, David Karp . . .

"Too much of the current discussion about the use and efficacy of psychiatric drugs proceeds from extreme, often ideologically based positions . . . To balance the picture we must learn how psychiatric patients themselves—the real

experts in their drama—try to make sense of what their prescribed medications do to them and for them."[14].

In my first consultations with Cornelia, she was very keen to know why I felt that Deanxit was not the right antidepressant for me, and she took what I said seriously, hence her decision to try to find something better for me. If she had thought my intuition, my opinion if you like, invalid, she would not have done so.

What was it, then, about Deanxit, that made me feel that it wasn't right for me? Firstly, I felt that it was enabling me to live life at a pace that I could not sustain, with negative impact on both myself and my family. I was in some senses, "better than well." And secondly, it had too negative an impact on the sexual side of my nature, which was putting an incredible burden on me. Either I had to give up sex, which didn't seem a solution at all, or I had to try to find a different antidepressant.

What about the antidepressant I'm on now, then? Since taking *Duloxetine* I have rediscovered the feeling of being sexually normal. It is, so far, unique in that it is not only a serotonin reuptake inhibitor, but also a *noradrenaline*, or *norepinephrine* reuptake inhibitor. Duloxetine contains my anxiety neurosis completely, *but* I remain aware of my limits, of my frailty. It does not make me "hyper", or give me such mood swings as Deanxit did. I'm actually *glad* to remain conscious of my frailty because this acts as a check on my natural enthusiasm, not dampening it, but enabling me to respect my limits. I will not dive head first into every idea or project that excites me, and believe me, there are many! My husband often remarks to people, somewhat wistfully, "Everything is Jane's favourite," or words to that effect.

With Duloxetine I feel *whole* somehow; it has restored my natural gifts and zest for life but without the crippling anxiety. It has enabled me to let go of my default function of wanting to control everything to avoid any unwanted surprises. This loss of anxiety has actually had quite a far-reaching effect on me.

Nevertheless, it came as a great surprise, and quite a disconcerting one in some ways, that my family said that I had changed. What did they mean? However, I don't think it was just the Duloxetine. During the somewhat cataclysmic year of 2010, I believe that God did something incredible for me in the realm of inner healing, and right in the midst of the crucible of suffering. So which was what? I don't know. I do know, though, that the inner healing started a good month before I started taking Duloxetine.

So, which is the real me; *with* the meds or without? My answer to that is, "both;" and then again, "neither", because all of us, as human beings, are both the same, and different people as we go through life—all of us without exception. We are recognizable, and yet different, with or without drugs. Transformation is a normal human phenomenon. As far as I can tell, apart from the change antidepressants have brought due to their neutralising severe anxiety, there are two other factors that are just as transformational in terms of character.

Enter cognitive psychology. In fact, I could have had a longer title to this book: Thank God for antidepressants *and* psychotherapy, because I wouldn't have been without either one, I needed them both.

Chapter 7
Little steps go a long way...

Inner rehabilitation

I had several periods of psychotherapy totalling about two years in all but spread out over twelve years; a first stretch of nine months, and then ten years later and for several years, several much smaller stretches.

The first occasion, back in 1985, is clearly etched in my mind. Manfred explained to me that we would see how it went, whether we each felt it was going somewhere and whether we clicked with each other. This was good, because it gave me a get-out, but it was a little threatening to me to think that it also gave Manfred a get-out! He also made it very clear that he himself, although being a doctor of psychology, also depended on God to enable him to discern "where to go." This struck me at the time as both reassuring and decidedly risky. What if God didn't make it clear to Manfred; what then? I needn't have worried!

Of course, I can no longer remember all the details of what we actually discussed, but I *do* remember clearly the questions that ran through my mind at that point: "How is he going to go about this? "What's the plan?" Being someone who felt a need for clear structure, it all seemed rather haphazard to me. And in a way it was, but

Jane Newman

this was actually its strength, as I was to learn, because this allowed things to emerge naturally. And emerge they did!

Our sessions, of one hour every two weeks, went something like this. We would chat about how life was going for me; what had happened recently, or something I remembered. Probably Manfred sparked it off with a question! Each time, in the conversation, he would put his finger on something, like the need to discover my protection in God rather than in controlling everything. This urge to control things sprung from fear and insecurity deep, deep down inside me. I wanted order, framework and predictability! Our children's school holidays were therefore a nightmare: no structure, no framework, and no predictability, especially with *four* children. I mean, with one television, how on earth could I cope with sorting out *which* child could watch *what*, and *when*? A sign-up rota helped a lot on that one!

Then at the end of our time, Manfred would suggest some practical step to take, kind of practical homework, rather like the exercises a physiotherapist gives you to correct something which is out of line, or out of condition. The old adage says, "Practice makes perfect". I would change that in this case to "practice makes it possible to change ingrained patterns and replace them with better ones." It was real, down to earth, *rehabilitation* of thought patterns and attitudes, because, as Professor Paul Gilbert puts it in his clear and compassionate book, "Overcoming depression," . . . .

. . . the way we think about things can itself be highly stressful.[15]

He points out how unconscious, core beliefs about ourselves and the world around us, often formed in childhood can skew our thinking and sabotage our family and social relationships. The *Cognitive Behavioural Techniques* approach aims to help us to "own" our needs and our motives, then challenge and, if necessary, replace our beliefs, expressed in our thoughts and words.

Manfred's approach, while being compatible with cognitive psychology, and in some ways appearing identical, aims elsewhere. His concern is to enable God's healing to reach us in the deepest part of our person. This is the part that influences our behaviour without our realizing it. With me, he often referred to the Bible to point out how God sees things, or what He is like. He then helped me to see how that could be worked out on the surface, walked out in the reality of life.

It was Manfred who introduced me to what he calls, "The art of taking little steps."[16] When he says "steps," he means practical actions you take in your everyday life, not high faluting theory. These actions, usually one per session, arose out of what we would have talked about: the "homework" mentioned above, to do for the next appointment. One example I clearly remember, was that the next time I asked my husband if he wanted to do something with me, like go for a walk, and that he replied "no, I'd rather do such-and-such", which I found very threatening, I should practice giving him the freedom to choose. Sure enough, before the next rendezvous came round, I had at least one occasion to put it into practice, and boy was it tough! Two things made it so; on the one hand, when John replied like that, I interpreted it to mean that he didn't love me, and on the other, I wasn't sure I wanted to let go of that and make the effort to really go for that walk on my own with the intention of enjoying it!

On another occasion, concerning my habit of automatically burying my emotions, Manfred encouraged me to try living more "on the surface," by which he meant; coming out with my feelings and expressing them, *as I was experiencing them*, rather than stifling them, which only meant them bursting out later in a delayed reaction from the depths of some subterranean emotional volcano. It boiled down to reducing the distance between the two parts of my person, the ideal being that they become integrated.

Now this was a big challenge for me. I first had to learn to recognize and name what I was feeling, which at first could take me days! Then I had to take what seemed to me the enormous risk of revealing them. And lastly I had to do it without dumping rubbish on the one whom I was addressing. There are of course really helpful techniques for learning this art, such as using "I", rather than the accusatory "you." Having become a past master at the skill of burying emotions I still have room for loads of improvement, and the hardest thing, is deciding to *come out with it*!

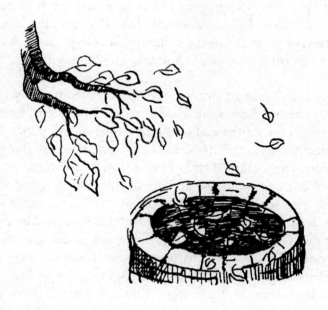

Keeping the well water clear from the little leaves
of insignificancies that float down each day . . .

Don't let the leaves sink to the bottom, but learn
to catch them as they settle.

But this is where Manfred's analogy of "little steps" is so helpful. I learned to see, and then congratulate myself for, every little step of improvement, rather than concentrating on the times I failed. It didn't take long for me to realize that I really was improving in this area, and that it made an enormous difference to my life, like walking free instead of lugging a heavy suitcase full of explosives that could go off any minute! (And they sometimes did!)

Over the course of two years of psychotherapy, as you can imagine, there were several more "little steps" that I worked on. At the end of the first nine-month period I remember saying to Manfred, "Look I'm due to give birth in one month's time, I feel like I've benefited enormously from our consultations, and I feel it would be good to stop." He replied along the lines of, "If it's enough for you for the moment, then it's enough for God, and its ok for me. God doesn't sort everything out in one go." So stop we did. Four months later, at the end of our year's sabbatical, we were once more back in the Ivory Coast, this time with three children. Although I had a bit of a rocky start back, finding my feet again in Africa and with a new baby, I didn't return to Manfred until nine years later, when I had several shorter courses of psychotherapy with him.

So maybe I could have made it with just psychotherapy, and no antidepressants? On that first occasion there was no question—I couldn't have. I needed the buoyancy of the medication to enable me to keep my head above water so that I could swim.

It was in 2012, twenty years later, that I came to wonder whether the inner rehabilitation that I had experienced was sufficient to warrant cutting out the antidepressants. After all, it would have been wonderful to witness to God's healing to this extent. It would be wonderful, too, not to have to remember to pack my medication every time I travelled; or on the other hand, not to experience the horror of realizing that I had forgotten it!

The six months' experiment of 2010 showed both Cornelia, my psychiatrist, and me that the answer was "No;" because even though I practised all I had learnt from psychotherapy, without medication I could not reap the benefits. I really *do* have something awry, or unbalanced, in my brain!

But God could heal that, couldn't he?

Chapter 8
Thank God?

The vexed question of healing
*". . . I am in a better place in my life now,
because of what I went through."*[17]

John Kirwan

And it is vexed, because we don't control it. We control it neither for ourselves nor for others, and on top of that, healing doesn't necessarily happen because all the right criteria have been fulfilled . . . if we even know what the right criteria are! Then if you add prayer into the mix, it still isn't a guarantee that you, or someone you pray for, will be healed.

Yes God could heal me so that I no longer need antidepressants. I'm convinced of that, because I've seen friends healed from all sorts of things, including cancer. But He hasn't; at least not yet. And He hasn't healed *all* my friends who battled with cancer. Some for whom I prayed, died, and they weren't elderly either. One friend died in her fifties leaving her husband and five children. Why?

I don't know. And for myself I don't *know*, either. Actually, at this point in time, I am so happy about the things he *has* healed me of, that I don't often think about it. Of course, if there were no Duloxetine to correct the deficiency, I most certainly *would* think about it, probably most of the time.

Having said that, I am ready to be surprised by God any time! I am reminded of Jennifer Rees Larcombe's honest and profound book, *Unexpected healing*. It still speaks to me of being ready for God to do the unbelievable, the unexpected. And probably do it in a most unorthodox way as he did for Jenny. First He arranged things such that a new, inexperienced Christian prayed for her healing when she was giving a talk at a conference. That's a little example of what the Apostle Paul called "the foolishness of God's wisdom!" After that, Jenny went to the bathroom and there, *in the bathroom*, she knew that she had to believe she had been healed and get up out of her wheelchair. And she did. Having come to terms with the fact she would never walk again, she suddenly found, as she took her first steps, that she could! Unexpected as it was to her, it was a total shock for her husband.

Yes, healing can be a vexed thing for nearest and dearest not only when it doesn't happen, but even when it *does* happen! Both circumstances require adjustment: emotional, physical and spiritual.

It may sound strange, but actually, I do see some benefits of *not* being healed of the need of antidepressants. That may sound shocking, bizarre, masochistic, whatever . . . but for me, it's true. It has been the means of my discovering Christ's love and His compassion that I feel fairly sure I never would have discovered had I stayed well, albeit handicapped without realizing it! Perhaps this is part of the justice of God? When He allows us to go through suffering, or trusts us with suffering, he comforts us, and we can't experience that comfort unless we suffer. Perhaps it is a law of life?

Now don't get me wrong! I have *never* wished to go through depression again in order to have more of this experience. Oh no! I'm no ethereal being untouched by earthly suffering. But I have found that when it does happen, it's actually not the end of the world. And yes, I discover more of myself, which is not always a pleasant thing, but it is salutary.

It has certainly made me question what we mean when we talk of healing, or when we pray for someone to be healed. In my case, the most obvious thing to pray was for me no longer to be in a state of needing antidepressants, to no longer be depressed. I did, very early on, have the experience of loving friends praying for me to be delivered of the depression. They came round one evening after supper and said they would only go when they had assurance that I had been delivered. This I found enormously stressful and not at all liberating! I felt rather that I had been put into a particular "box", where I didn't feel I belonged, and that I would only get out of it on their terms. It took them until midnight before they decided to go home; four chunks of eternity to me. I am so thankful to be able to say that this was the first *and* last of such experiences.

But what were my friends expecting? That God would wave a magic wand and not only heal me physiologically, but also of all my default behaviour patterns? I'm not saying He couldn't, but I do wonder if He would *choose* to do it that way because it's a question of habits, and processes, which happen over time. As for me, I certainly wouldn't want Him to stop at the physiological and not deal with the other things.

So what good do I see coming out of "the years that the locust has eaten" as one biblical writer put it? Were all those years of struggle wasted?

No, I don't believe they were. It was a strange thing at first, but I found that because I was vulnerable, others found it easier to confide in me about their sufferings. Not everyone, of course, but some. Those suffering from depression, and indeed other vulnerable conditions, felt I would be able to understand them, instead of being impatient, judgemental or blind to them.

Through depression, God has set things straight in my inner being that I didn't even realize were bent! And this has not only been good for me, but also for those around me!

John Kirwan puts it this way . . .

Depression is an experience that I would never play down. It's like a black hole, and it'll suck the life out of you if you don't get help. However, I'd also like to share with you, right at the beginning of this book, that in some ways having depression was a gift for me."[18]

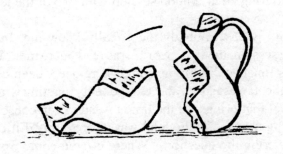

Broken, but not for the dustbin!

In these latter years, since 2009, He has healed me of a deep feeling of being somehow in exile, never at home; a sort of rootlessness. He started that during a week of something called "Wholeness through Christ." This is quite established in the UK and is becoming known in Switzerland. It is a most profound, healing experience. As a participant, you are prayed for by those conducting the week, and the other participants. Their prayers are in a form of listening to God and receiving "words" or pictures for you, like little messages really. These are noted down, moderated, and then those retained are given to you during an afternoon session with two of the team.

Now in my case, nobody there really knew me. In my private session, the first "word" was read out to me: "Your exile is finished." It hit me somewhere deep, deep down inside me. It was like an abscess suddenly bursting with all the relief that brings. At the time I wasn't even conscious of "being in exile," although I was aware of my difficulty in answering the question, "Where do you come from?" My reaction to this message was instantaneous; it took me totally by surprise. Tears welled up from within me and flowed freely: tears of joy and peace. It was an amazing moment. Two years later I was walking home from the train station, here in La Neuveville where I live, and as I looked up at the lower tower gate, the thought crossed my mind that I felt *at home* here. I felt I belonged. Now, that was *new*. It was like the healing had been walked out.

Two years later, when I got so sick while trying to find a more suitable antidepressant, I came to the point where one day I found myself thinking, "If this gets much worse, I could *die*." Now that's the kind of thought that gets your attention. It certainly got mine. But even though I was feeling terrible and had no concrete hope before me, I knew in that instant that I no longer feared death. In fact, I felt real joy at the thought of seeing Jesus. Boy! That was different! That wasn't me, was it?

Yes it was. Incredible though it seemed, it was. Not only had I always been afraid of my own death, I was very afraid of any of my children dying, would have regular nightmares about it; and I was also afraid of the time when my Mum and Dad would die. I just refused to consider it . . . the old burying instinct! Six months later my husband and I went to be with them for Christmas, and we realised that Mum was in her last months. I was able to accompany them through that time, and see my Mum off for Heaven, with *no fear*. Yes, I was sad, I missed her, and I found it difficult seeing her towards the end, looking so thin and just "hanging in there". But I was not afraid, I was happy for her to go *home*.

Another benefit I have gained through depression is freedom from trying to live up to others' expectations. When you hit rock bottom, when you can't get any lower, it somehow seems to pale into insignificance.

Depression has also given me the opportunity to take stock and reprioritize my life. I was stopped in my tracks, I was in some sense "still" and quite naturally thoughts, memories and insights rose up to the surface from deep within. It was a kind of "recueillement" as we say in French, and which can be translated as "collecting oneself, or collecting one's thoughts, or communing with oneself." To complete the process you need to listen to what rises up from within, take note, think about it, and then act.

I can recall quite vividly the moment when I realized that I was way too busy. I didn't have time to really "be present" with my children, or with the lady at the till in the supermarket. Every second was counted! I also realized that the guest studio I was running "on the side" of my mission and family work was actually taking up a lot of my time. I knew immediately that I wasn't meant to live life at such a frantic pace; neither did I *want* to do so. So I considered the guest studio work as a central part of what I did from that day on, along with the rest. It was counted, no longer just a little addition thrown in on the side. This enabled me to see more clearly what I needed to adjust in my life in order to slow down, and "be present".

This process of communing with oneself, of collecting one's thoughts, is such a necessary practice whether we are Christians or not.

Every person needs to know how to stop; to see clearly within them, to resist being driven by feelings, and to give back to our minds the control of our attitudes and behaviour. As the saying implies, the process consists in observing the disorder within one, and in putting things delicately back into place . . . Collecting oneself is precisely the place where choices are freely made.[19]

It is very different from fatalism, by which I mean shrugging your shoulders and saying, "nothing can be done;" as it is very different from the kind of meditation that gives momentary escape from reality. Collecting myself, or being connected to myself in the way I mentioned above set me on a path to places of choice and ultimately to thorough, fleshed out transformation.

As you will have maybe noticed in the preceding paragraphs, a lot of my help came from reading the Bible, especially meditating on it in a contemplative way. These moments are like a rendezvous with Jesus. We talk together, perhaps through the medium of reading a text from the Gospels recounting a particular event He lived. Sometimes, in the period when I was really sick, I was so tired I would drift off to sleep for a while right in the middle!

At other moments, I would have a thought pass through my mind, like someone was jogging my memory, which I believe He was! I have already recounted the "Job" thought. On another occasion, when I was feeling particularly devoid of hope, I recalled a song that had been sung at our Church retreat, "If you have faith, like a little grain of mustard, this is what the Lord says: 'You will be able to say to this mountain, pull yourself up and throw yourself into the sea!'" I recalled this at the bottom of the staircase, and I sang it out and stamped on each step as I made my way to the top! Suddenly I found myself in a different place, a place of courage and hope once more, with not a menacing mountain in sight!

But God didn't only come to my help through whispering me thoughts, or through words I read in the Bible. He helped me enormously through the few friends who were in the know, but perhaps not always in the way you might imagine! As I have already mentioned, they came on several occasions to help me pass the time in a way which would keep my focus off how sick I was feeling. They played scrabble with me! And they were each one so accepting of me, so *normal*. I'm so thankful to God for giving me friends like that. They are worth their weight in gold. Their company inhabited my loneliness and meant that my family did not need to carry the whole burden. But my family were great too. Special hugs, an invitation to lunch which meant I would eat properly, with a peaceful tummy, because I was in company . . . very practical things but which contributed hugely to my survival.

And of course, friends prayed. When I was in the eye of the storm, as Cornelia put it, she urged me to ask close friends to pray, which they did. I will never know in this life how much I owe to them. But I do know that just the fact of *knowing* they were praying was already helpful. I didn't feel alone in the fight.

Church services were more difficult because of the sheer number of people there—we have anything from sixty to a hundred people at services, or retreats, not to mention all the children. In earlier periods of depression I often drew a line through going to services. I didn't have the emotional strength for protracted conversations, challenging sermons or too many of the "How are you?" questions. However in 2010 I was able to attend most of the time, until I got too physically tired to do so, and I didn't have the same fear of facing many people.

I think the lack of fear was because I was much further down the road with antidepressants and had processed a lot of my ambiguous feelings about having to take them. I wasn't going to be fazed by someone else's remarks—unless of course they were hurtful, like the remark made to me at the end of a service, "well, haven't you *prayed* about it?" But you see, I've asked, I've been prayed for, I've been healed of a number of things which have brought me so much peace and freedom, and now I realize I need medication long term. It's part of a process of walking out my relationship with Jesus, of trusting Him even when I don't understand, keeping an open mind, and enjoying the peace of thankfulness.

I have made up my own mind where I stand, in the place of trust and thankfulness rather than the place of demanding healing or debating the question; which speaks of another huge area of healing that started way back in 1985 . . .

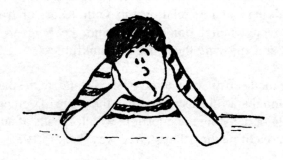

Decisions, decisions, decisions,
How I wish they would go away!
I can't cope with them today,
or any day.
Time to grow up, huh?
Ok, if to live means to choose, then I'll do it,
Even if it kills me![20]

Chapter 9
To live, is to choose[21]

It was probably 1986, I was on antidepressants and I knew I had to keep going another year until we could go on leave from Africa to Europe. One late afternoon, or it may have been morning,—I remember that the sun was hot—I set off down the dirt road that led from our administrative centre to the tarmac road and the shops of the Riviera 1 district in Abidjan. This was largely a residential neighbourhood with a few shops, lots of greenery and usually a pleasant breeze blowing off the lagoon which made it easier to bear the debilitating mix of heat and humidity.

I was off to the market stalls at the end of the dirt track to buy what I needed to make lunch. At siesta times I had been reading a book by Doctor Paul Tournier, *The Meaning of Persons*. In the midst of my deliberations on the theme of what I should cook for lunch, a chapter heading from the book simply barged in, unannounced: *To live is to choose*. It hit me forcibly right there that one of my major problems was that I did not want to choose. I did not want the responsibility of having to decide what we would eat for lunch, for example! It was too difficult and I recoiled from it even though I had no choice but to do it. Or did I?

At that moment, I realised something for the very first time. It is necessary to choose to do *even the things that you seem to have no choice over.* This kind of choosing could be translated by accepting willingly, even if one doesn't feel like it; or by owning your responsibility.

From that day on I accepted my task of being responsible for the family meals, whether I felt like it or not, and amazingly, that change in my attitude made the "weight" of decision-making much lighter. It still wasn't easy, but I wasn't adding resistance to the equation.

I didn't have access to any psychotherapy at the time, but reading Tournier's books was almost like having a session with a psychotherapist! His chapter heading stood out in large bold letters like they were dancing before my eyes, and they have been in some sense "with me" ever since.

Just a year ago, I realised that I had to go and confront a doctor who had been totally insensitive to one of my children. I didn't want to go at all. Until a couple of years ago I didn't *do* confrontation. In fact I would do all I could to *avoid* it. But I *chose* to do it even though I was scared and close to tears, because that chapter heading is still doing its work and enabling me to act like an adult and not a dependant.

Although such times are emotionally draining, especially so if you are going against your default way of functioning, not all choices are like that. Some are just a question of my getting up off my backside and getting on with something because it won't get done just by my wishing for it!

Of course, when it comes to big decisions, like antidepressants, *whether* and *which one,* it's good to have already practised on some smaller issues. And with antidepressants, as with many other things like sticking it out with one's life partner, or whether to be honest when one is in a system rife with corruption, the choice will probably not be made once and for all; not for me at any road.

Choosing is what makes us definite about something, intentional, committed . . . I think that's what Tournier means when he says that it's by choosing that you're really living. And the opposite is true too; not choosing is suffering life as a victim, and it's a real joy killer. The problem is that it can seem that someone who never gives their opinion or makes a suggestion is being very self-sacrificing and loving. I'm not so sure that it's always that. On the other hand, being positive and active doesn't mean fighting to have it all your own way, but rather being a vis-à-vis for the other, or others. You are giving them something to respond to. It calls out relationship and dialogue, while being on the defensive means things can just, well, peter out, lose their lustre or die.

I'll never forget the day in May 2010 when I asked Cornelia when I could go back to working full time. Her response absolutely gob-smacked me! She said something to the effect of: *Don't be in too much of a hurry to go back to work. It would be a pity to miss this opportunity to think about what you really want to do, whether you want to go on as before.* In that instant it hit me: I want to write! I even knew what I would write about first—because its message had been "in my suitcase" travelling with me through life, as it were, for many years—it just had never been fully unpacked. You guessed it; it's this book that you're reading right now!

But I didn't start writing it immediately. For a start, I wasn't well enough to do so. And then a few months later we moved house. So it wasn't until the summer of 2011 that it occurred to me that I needed to be *intentional* about this project, otherwise it just wouldn't happen. As any parent will no doubt agree, there's always enough to do on the home front to keep you busy, so if you don't set aside time for special projects, time flies past relentlessly and is lost.

I asked my friend, Danièle, if she would be a sounding board for me in the undertaking. I was mostly thinking of her reading the manuscript and giving comments from her psychotherapist's point of view. But Danièle did something even more important than that. She asked me what my deadlines were! When would I have written the first few chapters for her to read? Now *that* made me sit up straight! It got me going *and* over the inertia of fearing that I would *never* be able to write a chapter, let alone a book!

In a very real sense, I had to choose to believe in myself, and in the validity of the book. Many times along the way I doubted both, but encouraging comments from discerning friends and a positive professional appraisal of chapter 1 brought back the courage and determination. And I have loved it, all the way.

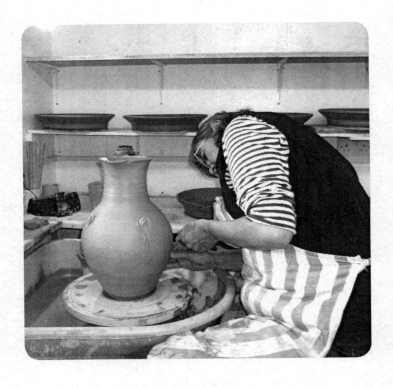

Louise potting

Chapter 10
Home

"God uses cracked pots,
and I'm the visual aid."[22]

The "I" in this context, is me. Then again, it could be anyone. Let me introduce you to Louise, my long time boarding-school friend.

Louise is a potter. She sells pottery to earn her living, but she also loves doing it. Now she recently gave me an oven dish she'd potted. "It's a second," she said apologetically, as she needed all the "firsts", the perfect ones, for her Christmas stall that she was rather frantically getting ready for after a period of ill health.

I just love that dish! I love its square shape, its dark brown colour, its size . . . I seem to want to use it for everything. But it's a second, because the colour didn't come out right: there are kind of rust-coloured spots on it. I actually even love the spots! And of course, it is mostly precious to me because it comes from her, and she is precious to me. But it really is a good dish!

Right then, when Louise gave it to me, it was like seeing a picture of God, the Master Potter[23]. There are several occasions related in the Bible where He is referred to as such, but as I'm beginning to expect, He doesn't do things the way I expect him to. He is so different, so much nicer, in a rather awe-inspiring way, than any of us can imagine! Instead of throwing me out, broken pot that I am, as "not good enough," He considers me precious, and has tenderly, carefully gathered up the pieces and mended me so that I may be not only a useful pot, but one He looks on with love and pleasure, rust spots and all!

I have already related how, from the first experience of depression, I was amazed to find that others who were feeling vulnerable could open up and talk to me when they knew that I was vulnerable too.

Gradually over the years I have grown in confidence that God can use this old cracked pot in ways I couldn't have imagined back then. To me, this is one of the most amazing things about the God of the Bible. He seems not to be fixed on brilliant performance but on *how* things are done; in trust, compassion and community.

I have also grown enormously in self-confidence because God *Himself* is "foolish enough" to trust in me. I'm not talking about *over* confidence, but rather a correcting of underlying *under* confidence. People who know me may be surprised by that because on the outside I give an impression of poise, strength and loads of confidence, but as Tournier puts it in his book, "The Weak and the Strong", what is strong can look weak, and what is weak can look strong.

However, this self-confidence does not at all mean that I feel light-hearted, or couldn't care less, about the fall out on my family from having a wife/Mum in depression. I have often felt guilty about it, and just as often fearful that they might face the same struggle in their lives. How will they cope? Will they find the right help? Not that such fear achieves anything useful, mind you.

I have given glimpses here and there in earlier chapters of the challenges thrown up for John and me as a couple by depression. Perhaps the major one is that of intimacy. If "the marriage act", as some have called it, was flawed, on my side (John insists that for him it didn't appear so,) for so many years, would that detract from intimacy, the feeling of togetherness, of closeness? Three things especially meant that this was not the case: baring our souls to one another; chucking out the ideal image of sexual love which we are fed relentlessly by books, films and television; and taking our marriage vows seriously.

I have a hunch that one of the main reasons there are so many divorces in the western world today is that we are being constantly fed a lie. Expressing love in a sexual way within a framework of faithfulness, or of marital covenant, is a challenge, a learning process and especially, a giving of one's whole being and in that sense, a sacrificial offering, and *not* a performance for which one gets marks out of ten! Anyhow, for us, once we had thrown out the lie, the pressure was off and we could concentrate on what really mattered.

There's no doubt that what nourished our intimacy enormously was the sharing of our thoughts, our hopes our disappointments, our feelings and our fears. This gave us a friendship and complicity, a secret garden of safety undergirding everything else. Not that this sharing

95

was easy, anything but, because there is always the fear that what you share, or the way you share it, might hurt the other irreparably. However, like many fears, this one turned out to be groundless. The contrary was the truth; by sharing our weaknesses, our love and complicity have been strengthened. This of course applies to any weakness we may be feeling, not just mental weakness.

And then there are the wedding vows. I still remember clearly that moment in the Church ceremony when we made ours. I shook! Just for half a second, but I wanted to mean what I said and the reality of the promise I made to John, especially the "for better *or for worse*" bit, definitely seemed more than I could be sure I could do. The enormity of it struck home. But I was counting on God, who invented marriage in the first place, to do His part! And John, going on what he has told me, must have been doing likewise. Today we are learning to rejoice *together* in our imperfections as we meet the challenges of growing older, slower and deafer!

I have had to learn in some sense to forgive myself, something I find a lot harder to do than to forgive others—that's pride! Actually, beyond forgiving myself, I have come to recognize that I couldn't do anything about the fall out: I had to trust God with that. I can pray for our children if they have to grapple with it, and of course, I can be understanding and try to offer that practical help and affection which I myself found so helpful. And most of all, I can *talk* with them about it, something I have not done well at all up to this point. Curiously it has been the writing of this book which has made me realize that this would be good to do. I also feel ready to do it now.

I'm not sure that I would have coped well two or three years ago.

I have also questioned whether John and I communicated in the best way on this issue with the children as they were growing up. Did we tell them enough? Did we tell them in a way they could understand? Did we tell them soon enough? The short answer is, "No." But this is not very helpful. It's like giving the score in a tennis match, 6-1, 6-4, 6-2, and saying it was a walkover when in fact nearly every game went to deuce and it was, in fact, hard fought!

In December 1997, I do have a clear memory of us sitting down with the children in our lounge, and John telling them that I wasn't well and would need their understanding and help. We didn't know at that stage what we do now, that it was going to turn out to be a long term condition, so we couldn't be much more precise; but maybe this was counterproductive and caused anxiety for them because it was so vague? Interestingly enough, none of our children remember our talking to them about it! And only our eldest realised that "something was amiss," but didn't know what it was.

What else, at that point in time, or later, could we have said? Maybe something like this; "Mum is going through a time where she is very, very anxious and not able to do as much as she usually does; it is called depression. It's not just ordinary worrying. It kind of makes her feel unable to do anything and makes her feel stressed out *all* the time. This makes her very tired and makes it hard for her to be flexible. She is taking medicine to help her with this, but it will take quite a while for her to feel better."

This book is at last giving me the opportunity of talking with them, and sharing with each of them in a way I haven't been able to before. It has actually brought me to the place of realising that I *owe* them such a time, to try to give them explanations, if they want any, and to answer *their* questions as best I can. They are all fully-fledged adults now, and on my side, I have a far greater understanding of depression in general, and my experience of it, than I had in earlier years. Indeed, in answer to the above questions, I'm not sure that we were in a place where we could have done a lot better, apart from the year when I was changing medication in 2010. At least at that point I could have given *something* in the way of an explanation, couldn't I? And yet it never occurred to me. I honestly don't think that I made a conscious decision *not* to. Maybe I was just too exhausted and too close to the experience to be able to do this? I think that's probably it.

But now I am so much looking forward to sharing with them whenever they feel ready to do so. I feel that this family fragility, stretching back at least as far as my two grandmothers, is at last losing its grip as it becomes faced, named, discussed, perhaps forgiven, and, hopefully, accepted. None of that will appear in this book. It is *their* story, not mine. I trust that with everything being completely open, they will be free from the burden of secrecy and shame. One of my sons told me he was proud of me. That is about the highest compliment and encouragement I could receive.

And that is where I am today, on the eve of my sixtieth birthday. From age thirty-three to sixty—that's been a long journey to freedom!

But . . .

- If the antidepressants I'm taking kill me sooner rather than later, but enable me to lead a meaningful, fulfilling life;

- If I can enjoy my marriage, my family and contribute to *their* lives in some positive way;

- If I can also be involved in serving others;

- And if on leaving this life what I will find will be immeasurably better . . .

What more do I want?

It's an important question to ask. It's one that I was able to ask *thanks* to depression, and *thanks* to the struggle to find the right antidepressant *for me*.

My answer is, "Nothing that I can think of right now."

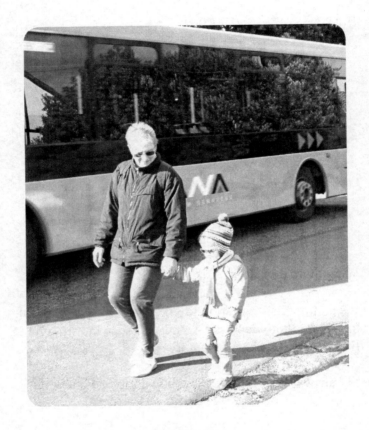

Travelling on

Postscript

And so life goes on. I will give my keyboard a rest, send the manuscript for proof-reading, and with my husband, get on a plane bound for New Zealand to see my brand new grandson. Then I am booked to go to England to accompany my ninety-two year old father on his move from Wiltshire down to Cornwall. A new chapter of life for all of us.

And then it will be back to my job, managing the web site of Wycliffe Switzerland. Back to our married son and his family, and our other two children—when they happen to drop by. Back to our little old town and our friends. Back to our apartment above our doctor's surgery and next to the motorbike shop, with its lake-view balcony exposed to three of the four winds and to daylong sunshine—sometimes!

Then on again . . . towards retirement and a new chapter for John and me, and maybe into the next two books which have been simmering on the back burner for a whole year! They are quite different in nature, one being on "Cooking to combat digestive candida . . . cheerfully" and the other on learning the forgotten art of contemplation in our reading of the Bible. I'm looking forward to it immensely.

Bibliography

Engeli, Manfred 2007. *Makarios, ou en route pour le Bonheur.* Dossiers Vivre

Gilbert, Paul 2000. *Overcoming depression.* Constable and Robinson, London.

Karp, David 2007. *Is it me or my meds?* First Harvard University Press.

Kirwin, John, October 2010. *All blacks don't cry.* Penguin, New Zealand.

Maire, Charles-Daniel 2009. *Identité subie ou identité choisie?* Olivétan, Lyon.

Rees Larcombe, Jennifer 1991. *Unexpected Healing.* Hodder & Stoughton.

Tournier, Paul 1976. *The Strong and the Weak.* The Westminster Press, Philadelphia.

Tournier, Paul 1957. *The Meaning of Persons.* Buccaneer Books, New York. Ch.11.

Websites

www.depression.co.nz

John Kirwan' site. Although contact links are for New Zealand, this is a brilliant resource for anyone understanding English, wherever they live.

Endnotes

¹ New Oxford Dictionary of English, OUP 2001.

² Doctor Paul Tournier was a pioneer in what was called *Medicine of the person.*

"Medicine of the Person" is not just another branch of medicine. "It is an attitude towards contact, an approach to patient-care, applicable in all areas. It puts the emphasis on awareness of patients as whole persons, with places in their community and society. Both the organic and the psychological approach are integral parts of Medicine of the Person, as is consideration of the connection between state of health, life events, social insertion and spirituality."

Tournier's books, see the Bibliography, were like fire-side companions to me during the worst years of depression, and life-changing effects on me through his telling of real stories, his own and those of his patients. I cannot recommend them more highly.

³ Flanders and Swann, *At the drop of another hat,* 1963.

⁴ Aloe Vera drinking gel, virtually pure Aloe Vera, is particularly good for clearing urinal tract infections. The Gel Concentrate is excellent for vaginal application during and after menopause to keep the flora in balance, often a cause of Urinal tract infections. You need to obtain these products from reputable companies like "Forever", or "LR World".

⁵ Jane Newman, *Fragments,* 1993 SIL Abidjan, out of print

107

6   John Kirwan, *All Blacks never cry*: October 2010 Penguin. See also: http://www.allblacksdontcry.com/wordpress/ for a free viewing of the film based on the book, and for all the comments.

7   David A. Karp—*is it me or my meds?*—Living with antidepressants, p.102. See the case of Sarah.

8   Paul Gilbert, *Overcoming depression,* 2000 Constable and Robinson, p.ix, Foreword.

9   *The Week*: October 22nd 2011

10 Jane Newman, *Fragments,* 1993 SIL Abidjan, out of print.

11 The Bible. *Paul's letter to the Corinthians*, chapter 5, verse 17. Good News Bible.

12 Paul Gilbert, *Overcoming depression,* 2000 Constable and Robinson, p.65.

13 David A. Karp—*is it me or my meds?*—Living with antidepressants.

14 David A. Karp—*is it me or my meds?* Living with antidepressants, P.17

15 Paul Gilbert, *Overcoming depression,* 2000 Constable and Robinson, P.367.

16 Manfred Engeli, *Makarios, ou en route pour le bonheur.* Dossiers Vivre, 2007, Appenix.

17 John Kirwan, *All Blacks never cry*: October 2010 Penguin. P. 12.

18 John Kirwan, *All Blacks never cry*: October 2010 Penguin. P. 12.

19 Charles-Daniel Maire, *Identité subie ou identité choisie?* Olivétan, 2009, pp. 149 and 150, translation mine.

20 Jane Newman, *Fragments,* 1993 SIL Abidjan, out of print.

21 Paul Tournier, *The meaning of persons*, 1957 Buccaneer Books, New York, Ch 11.

22   Patsy Clairmont, the title of a talk that a friend of mine had recorded and passed on to me to enjoy; and enjoy it I did!

23   The Bible. *Jeremiah* chapter 18, verse 4, and Psalm 31 verses 9 and 12 for example.

Lightning Source UK Ltd.
Milton Keynes UK
UKOW040211061012

200144UK00005B/1/P